Mini Mixing Manual

by

The Natural Maven

Copyrights

Mini Mixing Manual by The Natural Maven

Published by Raw Digits Media Group

Jacksonville, Florida

www.DuvalTheMusical.com

© 2018 Christavia Dickinson

ISBN:978-1983739545

Table Of Contents

Preface...5

Toxins in Products.................................7

Benefits of Using Organic Products..................9

Quick Tips...11

Hair Care..13

Skin Care..27

Remedies...37

Glossary...55

Write Your Own Recipes............................85

Supply List/Notes.................................91

Conversion Chart..................................95

Raw Beauty Pledge.................................96

I dedicate this book to my grandmother,

Who taught me how to wait and pray

Who taught me a more simple way

I love you and I know you would be proud today

Preface

I created this mini manual to provide a healthier alternative to commercial products and our lifestyle habits. Commercial products can contain cancer causing ingredients and they are not good for our hair or skin. As a cosmetologist, I have seen the irreversible damage that toxic products can cause so I am on a mission to bring awareness to this ongoing but unchallenged issue.

Remember this book is just a guideline! The combinations of mixing possibilities are endless. Once you begin to find success in your mixing, you will realize that you can change any recipe formulation to fit you perfectly. So try a recipe, reformulate it and try it again!

Come with Me

I wasn't always the type to care about the wellness of

humanity

I used to be a selfish and lonely person who couldn't

see past their self

I used and abused my body in so many ways

Until I broke down and said,

"I am tired of this destructive life!"

I knew it wasn't right

I knew it was time for a lifestyle change

A change that would renew my life

A change that relieved my financial strife

I hope that you can see the reasons to join me

On this inspirational natural journey!

Toxins in Products

The majority of Americans are not familiar with genetically modified organisms, but GMOs are in 80% of the processed foods and beauty products in our local stores. These organisms do not occur naturally but are created in a laboratory by scientist to enhance our products. GMOs have been banned due to reports of sickness and environmental damage in other developed countries like Europe, Australia and even Japan. The United States has decided not to ban these organisms because the organisms have been tested and labeled as safe by the same company who creates the organisms. Companies who create these organisms are placing them in all their products without sharing the knowledge with the public.

Most people have no idea how these toxic products effect their daily lives because they do not experience immediate effects. Harmful toxins are being found in our water, food, cosmetics, clothes, air and medicines but we continue to pay major companies for more toxic products because we have become familiar with them.   Almost all American families have experienced some sort of loss due to cancer in themselves or a close family member yet many still do not eliminate or correct the cause.

We may not be able to eliminate all the harmful chemicals in our environment, but our health will benefit greatly from small changes implemented in our daily lives.

Benefits of Using Natural Products

While some toxic products meant for consumption are cheaper than their all-natural alternatives most are more expensive. For example, when comparing a commercial bottle of foam to natural flax seed gel, a seven-and-a-half-ounce bottle of commercial foam costs about fifteen dollars and yields about seven uses. A sixteen-ounce bag of flax seeds cost about ten dollars and yields about sixteen uses. In this scenario, the flax seeds are five dollars cheaper for more than twice the amount of commercial foam product.

Product companies benefit tremendously by creating elaborate product lines that supposedly work in conjunction with each other. These product lines cause consumers to purchase more products with the belief that they can achieve better benefits by buying additional products from the product line. Major hair product companies are mostly guilty for pushing this marketing tactic and it creates confusion for many customers. They are normally left wondering how many products to buy and exactly how to use the manufactured combination. When using natural products, most have multiple uses, so you use less products to achieve the same or better results.

The most beneficial benefit of using natural products is that you can add or remove whatever you like or dislike. If you buy a shampoo for your local hair store and are not satisfied with it, you can not go back to the store and ask them to remake it to your liking. With natural alternatives, you can adjust each recipe to accommodate your needs until you find the perfect formula.

Base oils are oils that are used to dilute essential oils. They are normally mixed in larger quantities in formulations.

Common Base Oils: Olive, Grapeseed, Coconut, Avocado, Sunflower, Jojoba, Almond, Sesame

Essential oils are potent oils made from parts of beneficial plants in our environment. These oils carry a variety of benefits based on the plant's healing properties. These oils are mixed in smaller quantities and are usually measured in drops. Find our list of essential oils in our glossary.

- Mix your formulas starting from the largest quantity moving to the smallest to ensure even mixing.

- Some formulas require refrigeration to extend the shelf life.

- Most mixtures will have to be shaken or stirred before every use.

- Some ingredients mix better when warm.

- While in the trial phases of formulating we suggest that you use smaller portions until you find your perfect formula

- You can also change the base oil to fit your hair or skin type.

You will find natural alternatives for every hair product you use in this manual. Feel free to add or remove whatever you want. Remember these products are completely organic so they may not look like the homogeneous mixture that you are used to, but they work wonders!

To achieve the best formulations, you must know your hair type. The four hair types are straight, wavy, curly and kinky. Straight and wavy hair formulations should include less oils and more volumizing ingredients. Curly and kinky hair must use heavier oils and deep moisturizing ingredients. To learn more about the health of your hair visit us online or call your local cosmetologist.

Don't know your hair type? Try this simple hair type test. While your hair is wet, pull a piece of hair from the back of your hairline and compare it to the image below.

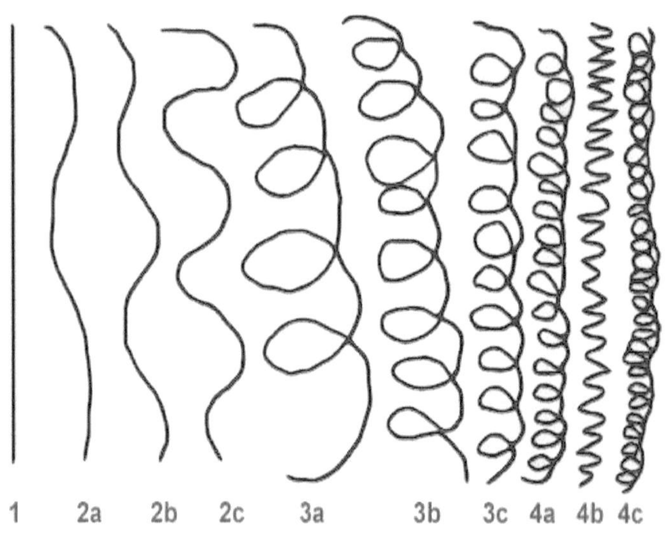

Flax Seed Gel

3 cups water

1/3 cup flax seeds

knee high stocking or cheesecloth

small pot

mixing bowl

storage jar

gloves (optional)

Put water and flax seeds in a small pot. Bring water to a boil on medium high heat. Stir frequently. Keep boiling until water begins to turn into a jelly like texture (about five to seven minutes). Allow to cool. Put the knee high in the storage jar and secure the band around the jar lid. Pour flax seed gel into stocking. Pick up stocking and place into mixing bowl. Squeeze out all the gel until you see a white foam. Throw away the stocking. Pour gel into storage container. Refrigerate. Gel may be kept for seven days. Makes about one cup of gel. If you want a different consistency to your gel, you can make your gel thicker by using less water and more flax seeds or thinner by adding more water and less flax seeds.

Hair Growth Serum

½ cup onion juice

1 cup castor oil

1 teaspoon cayenne pepper powder

1 teaspoon cinnamon powder

7 drops lavender oil

container

Mix onion juice and castor oil. Stir in cayenne and cinnamon. Add lavender and stir briskly. Apply to affected areas. Massage area for ten minutes. Allow to sit for at least thirty minutes then shampoo and condition. Use peppermint shampoo for an extra boost!

1 pound shea butter

2 ounces raw beeswax

3 tablespoons vegetable glycerin

½ cup olive oil

½ cup coconut oil

small pot

storage container

Place beeswax in a small pot and melt to liquid on low heat. Once liquefied, add shea butter and allow to melt. Mix frequently. Once liquefied, remove from heat. Add coconut and olive oil, then stir in vegetable glycerin. Allow to cool then transfer to storage container. Shelf life is up to 6 months. Best for thicker hair or color damaged hair.

Edge Control

3 teaspoons flax seed gel

1 teaspoon honey

pinch of xanthan gum

Mix xanthan gum with honey. Stir briskly to ensure gum is evenly mixed. Stir in flax seed gel until evenly mixed. Apply product with your fingers and/or a soft brush to control your unruly hairs along your hairline. Refrigerate any unused portion. Use within seven days. If any mold forms, discard immediately.

Hydrating Oil

3 tablespoons olive oil

1 tablespoon avocado oil

1 tablespoon coconut oil

1 tablespoon argan oil

small container

Mix all oils in a storage container. You can apply it to your scalp and hair with your fingers or a squeeze bottle. Increase your hydration by covering your hair with a plastic cap after applying oil. Use a blow dryer to apply heat to the cap for at least five minutes.

Conditioner

1 cup mayonnaise

essential oils (optional)

small bowl

Put mayo in a small bowl. Mix with essential oils that benefit your hair and scalp conditions. Apply conditioner to hair from root to ends and allow the mixture to penetrate your hair for at least thirty minutes. Rinse out with lukewarm water, dry and style as usual.

Shampoo

1 cup castile soap (any type)

1 cup distilled water

13 drops essential oils

empty shampoo bottle

Pour water, castile soap and essential oils into your empty shampoo container. Shake vigorously. Use shampoo as you would with manufactured shampoo. Do not expect your first shampoo to lather much. For best results, shampoo twice and use warm water.

1 teaspoon grapeseed oil

1 teaspoon sunflower oil

Mix oils evenly. Apply a very small amount (smaller than an American dime) to the ends of freshly shampooed or damp hair. Massage oil into your hair from the root to the ends. Blow dry hair on low heat. Style as usual. Never apply this mixture to dry hair because it will weigh your hair down.

Stimulating Oil

1 tablespoon base oil

7 drops peppermint oil

3 drops tea tree oil

container

Pour base oil into a container. Add the peppermint and tea tree oils. Mix evenly. Apply to areas that need to be stimulated. Massage the area in a circular motion for ten to fifteen minutes twice a day.

Volumizer

2 sixteen-ounce beers (room temperature, extra hops)

3 ripe bananas

3 teaspoon olive oil

mixing bowl

Mash up bananas and olive oil in mixing bowl. Add in 1/3 cup of beer and mix evenly. Add banana mixture to hair from root to end. Cover hair with a plastic cap and wear for at least 30 minutes. Rinse hair with warm water until mixture is removed. Rinse hair with the remaining beer and let sit for ten minutes. Rinse lightly. Blow dry hair upside down for maximum volume.

Skin Care Recipes

Our skin care section has everything for your daily specialized skin care regimen. To achieve radiant skin you should always cleanse, exfoliate, tone, mask and moisturize with product specific for your skin type. There are four main skin types: normal, dry, oily and combination skin. Normal skin is balanced and does not have any major skin conditions. Dry skin does not produce enough sebum, or oil. Oily skin over produces sebum and combination skin is a combination of dry and oily skin. Whatever skin type you may have, it is not impossible to attain great skin!

Don't know your skin type? Try this simple skin test!

After waking up, gently pat your face in small sections with a piece of cosmetic blotting paper. Use one paper for each area of the face: chin, cheeks, forehead and nose. Hold the paper up to a light and examine the amount of oil on the paper. If the paper has excessive oil on it from all areas of the face you have oily skin. If the paper does not have any or only a little oil from all areas of the face, you have dry skin. If your blotting papers only have oil on the nose and forehead area, you have combination or normal skin. For more detailed skin analysis, visit your local esthetician.

Funny Fact

Your skin is the largest organ of your body!

Deodorant Bar

1 ounce beeswax

2 tablespoons coconut oil

1 tablespoon arrowroot powder

13 drops essential oil

one teaspoon baking soda (optional)

small candy mold

small sauce pan

Melt beeswax in a small sauce pan on low heat. Stir frequently. Once liquefied, stir in coconut and essential oil (stir in baking soda). Pour mixture into candy mold while hot. Allow up to 30 mins to cool. Use in any sweaty area to combat body odors. Perfect for children!

Skin Moisturizer

1/4 cup vegetable glycerin

1/4 cup jojoba oil

1/4 cup hemp oil

storage container

Pour oils into container and mix thoroughly. Apply to skin while damp for best results. Use a towel to pat away an excess oils from your skin. You can also try adding a few drops of your favorite essential oil to increase its benefits.

Toner

2 teaspoons lemon juice

1 teaspoons honey

1 teaspoons base oil

small container

Pour lemon juice, honey and base oil into the container. Mix thoroughly. Use your fingertips, a small paint brush or foundation brush to apply the mixture to your face. Massage into skin using small circular upwards motion. Gently pat off excess toner with a cool wet rag or hand towel. Do not rub your face. Discard unused portion.

Sugar Scrub

1 cup cane sugar

1/2 cup base oil

7 drops essential oil

small bowl

Pour cane sugar into a small bowl. Mix in base and essential oils until the sugar looks slushy. Moisten the skin, preferably with a steamy towel, before exfoliating. Rub the sugar scrub in circular motions for at least three minutes. Rinse the area with warm water to remove excess sugar and oil. Pat skin dry with a towel.

Detox Mask

3 tablespoons bentonite clay

1 tablespoon activated charcoal

3 tablespoons water

small bowl

paint or foundation brush

Pour bentonite clay and activated charcoal into small bowl and mix evenly. Slowly mix in water. Consistency should be like a thin paste. Use your brush to apply the mask to your skin. Allow to dry and sit for at least thirty minutes. Rinse mask off with a warm dark colored washcloth.

Lip Balm

1 ounce beeswax

1 tablespoon jojoba oil

3 drops essential oil

small sauce pan

small candy mold or container

Place beeswax in small saucepan and melt on low heat. Once liquefied, stir in jojoba and essential oils. Remove from heat. Pour mixture into mold and allow to cool. If using a container, allow to cool then transfer lip balm to your container.

Deodorizing Salt Soak

1 cup epsom salt

7 drops dill oil or 1/3 cup dill leaves

7 bay leaves

Gather all ingredients before preparing hot water for soaking. Once hot water is prepared, pour Epsom salt, dill oil and bay leaves into the water. Allow water to sit for at least 10 minutes. Soak the affected area for at least fifteen minutes.

Herpes Healer

1 tablespoon olive oil

13 drops Melissa oil

7 drops neem oil

3 drops vanilla (optional)

small bowl

Combine all ingredients into a small bowl. Mix thoroughly. Apply a small amount to the affected area twice to three times a day. Mostly used for common cold sores on the lip.

All-Natural Remedies

Our remedies section has some of grandma's old tricks as well as a few more tips. You will find everything from fever reducers, natural home cleansers and even a healthy homemade dog food recipe. When using your natural remedies remember consistency is key! Use your remedy for at least three to seven days for best results.

All Purpose Cleaner

16 ounces water

3 drops lemon oil

3 drops tea tree oil

spray or squeeze bottle

Pour water into your spray bottle. Pour in essential oils. Shake vigorously. Spray soiled areas. Wipe with a clean cloth. Works great on most surfaces especially in bathrooms and kitchens!

Insect Repellent

1 gallon water

1 cup lemongrass

½ cup rosemary

15 drops lemon oil

30 drops neem oil

15 drops orange oil or any citrus oil

strainer

heavy duty spray bottle

crock pot

Pour water into crock pot and turn on high. Add remaining ingredients. Stir. Allow mixture to simmer overnight. Let cool. Strain mixture. Pour mixture back into gallon jug. Spray the insect repellent anywhere and allow to air dry.

Mucus Relief Bath

1 cup basil leaves

3 sliced or diced onions

1 cup oregano

30 drops eucalyptus

15 drops frankincense

bathtub filled with hot water

cheese cloth

Fill bathtub with hot water. Lay cheese cloth flat but keep it folded so that you can not see through it. Add ingredients to the center of the cheese cloth and secure it tightly. Place the ball of herbs in the bathtub and allow to sit for at least ten minutes. Get into the bathtub and soak for at least fifteen minutes. While soaking, take deep breaths and place the herbs on your chest for maximum results.

2 cups baking soda

16 ounces white vinegar

spray bottle

Pour vinegar into spray bottle. Sprinkle baking soda on the area that needs to be cleaned. Spray the area with your vinegar bottle. Allow mixture to sit for at least three minutes. Scrub surface with an abrasive cleansing pad. Rinse area with hot water.

Refresher Pads

cotton ball or rounds

7 drops lemon oil

7 drops essential oil of your choice

Saturate the cotton with the essential oils. Place in areas that need refreshing like bathrooms, garbage cans and diaper pails. You can also add in additional citrus oils like grapefruit and orange.

1 gallon water

½ cup thyme

½ cup rosemary

13 bay leaves

13 drops peppermint oil

20 drops lemon oil

strainer

crock pot

Put gallon of water in the crock pot. Turn crock pot to high. Add the remaining ingredients to the crock pot. Allow to simmer overnight. Let cool. Strain mixture. Use a spray or squeeze bottle to apply mixture to pet. Allow to air dry.

Detox Drink

2 teaspoons activated charcoal

3 tablespoons honey

1 teaspoon lemon juice (optional)

8 ounces water

small pot

Pour water into pot and simmer on medium heat. Pour activated charcoal and honey into a cup. Add the hot water to the cup and stir briskly until honey is dissolved. Stir while drinking to ensure that you drink the charcoal. While detoxing your body make sure that you drink plenty of water.

1 tablespoon olive oil

1 teaspoon cayenne pepper

7 drops peppermint oil

small bowl

Combine all the ingredients into a bowl. Mix evenly. Apply directly to the area of the head that hurts the most. Massage for at least five minutes. Allow solution to sit for up to thirty minutes. Remove solution with a cool towel. Ensure that the solution doesn't come in contact with any cuts or your eyes.

Teeth Whitener

1 tablespoon activated charcoal

toothbrush

Wet your toothbrush with water. Cover your toothbrush with the charcoal. Brush your teeth for at least 2 minutes. Rinse charcoal completely from your mouth. Use this remedy for at least three but no more than seven days consecutively for a brighter smile.

1/2 tablespoon sesame oil

1/2 tablespoon coconut oil

small bowl

Mix oils into a small bowl. Pour oils into your mouth. Pull the oils through your teeth for up to twenty minutes. Spit out oil. Rinsing with water is optional. You can also add your favorite flavored essential oil for a more enjoyable experience.

Pressure Reducer

1 tablespoon apple cider vinegar

1 teaspoon turmeric

1 teaspoon sesame oil

3 tablespoons honey

8 ounces water

small pot

Pour water into your pot and turn on medium heat. In a cup, add the remaining ingredients. Once water is warm, pour into the cup. Stir until all ingredients are dissolved. Drink mixture anytime, up to three times a day. This can also be beneficial to people with diabetes and high cholesterol.

7 drops clove oil

7 drops lime oil

cotton swab

small bowl

Combine both oils into a small bowl. Mix oils with swab. Use the swab to generously apply oils onto the affected areas. You can also substitute the lime oil for extra clove oil.

Air Freshener

8 ounces warm water

1 cup vanilla extract

3 tablespoons nutmeg

spray bottle

Mix all ingredients into your spray bottle. Shake
vigorously. Spray in areas where refreshing is needed.
Great for removing odors from beds, couches and
pillows!

parsley leaves

13 drops peppermint oil

7 drops lemon oil

pestle and mortar

Put parsley leaves in the mortar. Add the essential oils to the parsley leaves. Use the pestle to grind the ingredients. Chew the mixture anytime, to battle bad breath. Spitting out parsley leaves is optional. Try adding a pinch of cane sugar for a sweeter taste.

Wrinkle Reducer

1 pound shea butter

1/2 cup olive oil

1/2 cup sunflower oil

1/4 cup sage

10 drops lime oil

small pot

Put shea butter in a small pot. Melt on medium heat. Stir frequently. Add remaining ingredients and mix thoroughly. Simmer for at least ten minutes. Allow to cool down. Pour mixture into a container. Use on affected area at least twice a day for best results.

Dog Food

1 cup of chicken (boneless, cooked)

1 cup of salmon

1 tablespoon mixed vegetables

1 tablespoon kidney beans (optional)

Mix all ingredients. Serve your pet in serving sizes acceptable for their weight. When feeding your dog beans, there will be an increase in bowel movements so feed on occasion. Never cook your dog's food with seasoning, it can be detrimental to their health!

Glossary

The International Phonetic Alphabet is a system created by linguist that shows others how to pronounce a word with special characters. The system is elaborate and filled with symbols that are not common to the English language. To make these words easier to understand and pronounce we have included the phonetic spelling and syllable breakdown of each word to help you pronounce them. In the syllable breakdown there may be a **bold** syllable. This syllable will be stressed or said a little louder and longer than the other syllables.

Example word- apple

[**ap**-uhl] Phonetic Spelling

[ˈ**æp**-əl] IPA

A

Apple cider vinegar [**ap**-uhl **sahy**-der **vin**-i-ger]

Detoxifying, relieves diabetes symptoms,

prevents dandruff, lowers blood pressure, helps

weight loss, decongestant, increases energy,

improves circulation

Aloe [**al**-oh]

Heals skin conditions, relieves constipation,

helps with breathing problems, anti-

inflammatory

Avocado [ah-vuh-**kah**-doh]

Helps with weight management, protects skin

from aging, antioxidant, heals psoriasis,

moisturizes

Argan oil [**ar**-gen oil]

Hydrates and softens skin and hair, reduces

frizz, antioxidant, prevents stretch marks

Activated charcoal [**ak**-tuh-vey-ted **chahr**-kohl]

Detoxifies, prevents hangovers, lowers

cholesterol, whitens teeth, treats burns, gas and

bloating

Almond oil [**ah**-muhnd oil]

Treats cholesterol and cardiovascular disease,

reduces diabetes symptom, promotes weight

loss

Arnica oil [**ahr**-ni-kuh oil]

Reduces pain, swelling and stiffness, heals

bruises, promotes hair growth

Arrowroot [**ar**-oh-root]

Balances pH in body, used as an alternative for

baby powder and breast milk, heals skin

conditions, mild laxative, deodorizer

B

Bentonite clay [**ben**-tn-ahyt kley]

> Absorbs toxins, helps with intestinal problems,
> soothes skin allergies

Bay leaves [bey leevz]

> Treats arthritis, insomnia, reduces pain,
> antibacterial, antifungal, helps respiratory
> problems

Bergamot [**bur**-guh-mot]

> Refreshing, uplifting, treats anxiety, depression,
> antibiotic, antiseptic, helps digestive system

Basil [**baz**-uhl]

> Clarifying, aids in concentration, anti-
> inflammatory, combats cells, helps heart health

Beeswax [**beez**-waks]

> Protects skin from irritants, anti-inflammatory,
> antibacterial, antiviral

Baking soda [**bey**-king **soh**-duh]

> Relieves digestion issues, kills mold, fungi and
> parasites, reduces coughing and sore throat

Black pepper [blak **pep**-er]

> Treat pain, reduces fever, improves circulation,
> aids in digestion, anti-inflammatory, antioxidant

Birch [burch]

> Treats depression, antiseptic, astringent, repels
> insects, disinfectant, relieves urinary issues

Black walnut oil [blak **waul**-nuht oil]

> Antifungal, antimicrobial, combats cancer cells,
> increases cardiovascular strength, expels
> parasites

C

Citronella oil [si-truh-**nel**-uh oil]

> Repels insects, antiseptic, anti-inflammatory, reduces depression, antibacterial, kills worms in intestines

Cinnamon [**sin**-uh-muhn]

> Antimicrobial, anti-inflammatory, relieves depression, aphrodisiac, kills parasites, increases immunity

Cassia [**kash**-uh]

> Improves circulation, anti-inflammatory, treats menstrual symptoms, relieves constipation and coughing

Clary sage [**klair**-ee seyj]

> Aphrodisiac, antidepressant, regulates menstrual cycles, astringent, sedative, improves digestion

Camphor [**kam**-fer]

> Decongestant, disinfectant, anti-inflammatory,
>
> relieves pain, antifungal, increases circulation

Cannabis flower oil [**kan**-uh-bis **flou**-er oil]

> Powerful stress and pain reliever, boost appetite,
>
> skin protectant, aids in digestion, prevents some
>
> types of cancer (may be illegal in some areas)

Carrot seed oil [**kar**-uht seed oil]

> Treats damages skin, relieves pain, moisturizes
>
> and naturally tans skin, increases appetite

Cumin [**koo**-muhn]

> Aids in digestion, antiseptic, increases immunity,
>
> helps with insomnia, antiviral, rejuvenates skin

Cane sugar [keyn **shoog**-er]

> Exfoliates dead skin cells, unrefined sugar,
>
> includes antioxidants

Chamomile [**kam**-uh-meel]

> Calming, refreshing, sedative, antidepressant, treats infections and head lice

Coconut oil [koh-kuh-nut oil]

> Conditions hair, prevents cardiovascular disease and high blood pressure, anti-inflammatory, boost immune system

Castor oil [**kas**-ter oil]

> Improves immunity, induces labor, increase circulation, promotes hair growth, anti-inflammatory, relieves constipation

Cocoa butter [**koh**-koh **buht**-er]

> Moisturizes skin, increases immune system, antioxidant, relieves skin conditions, reduces cardiovascular issues

Cedarwood [**see**-der-wood]

> Sedating, strengthening, promotes healthy skin, treats eczema and other skin conditions

Cypress [**sahy**-pruhs]

> Astringent, relaxing, mosquito repellent, fights infection, detoxify, treats anxiety

Clove [klohv]

> Kills insects, relieves tooth aches, respiratory issues, antiseptic, reduces stress, prevents premature ejaculation

Cayenne [kahy-**en**]

> Detoxifies, stimulates hair growth, aids in digestion, reduces migraines and cramps, lowers cholesterol levels

D

Dill [dill]

Helps with digestion, antioxidant, calming, disinfectant, sedative, relieves muscle spasms

E

Eucalyptus [yoo-kuh-**lip**-tuhs]

Decongestant, antiseptic, treats dandruff, cooling, repels insects

Epsom   salt [**ep**-suhm sawlt]

Relieves muscle pain, relaxing, reduces stress, detoxifying, treats constipation, improves circulation

Evening primrose oil [**eev**-ning **prim**-rohz oil]

Reduces PMS, pain, increases fertility, relieves skin conditions, treats osteoporosis

Flax seed [flaks seed]

> Superfood, reduces diabetes, strokes and heart disease, combats cancer cells, anti-inflammatory, holds hair in place

Fennel [**fen**-l]

> Relief from gas and indigestion, increases milk production, treats osteoporosis, lowers blood pressure, prevents cancer

Frankincense [**frang**-kin-sens]

> Dispels fears, eases breathing, helps with meditation, increases immunity, astringent, balances hormones

Fenugreek [**fen**-yoo-greek]

> Helps with digestion, relaxing, fights infection, increases milk production, antioxidant, anti-inflammatory

Fish oil [fish oil]

> Reduces cardiovascular disease, lowers blood
> pressure, promotes weight loss, improves eye
> sight, anti-inflammatory,

Fir needle oil [fur **need**-l oil]

> Fights infections and odor, treats arthritis and
> muscle pain, relieves sore throat, combats
> cancer causing cells

G

Ginger [**jin**-jer]

> Fights common cold and respiratory problems,
> treats nausea, anti-inflammatory, helps digestive
> issues

Grapeseed oil [**greyp**-seed oil]

Lowers cholesterol, light moisturizer for skin
and hair, lubricant, seals hair cuticles, anti-
inflammatory, reduces wrinkles

Geranium [ji-**rey**-nee-uhm]

Balancing, harmonizing, antibacterial,
antimicrobial, anti-inflammatory, reduces acne

Grapefruit oil [**greyp**-froot oil]

Toner, purifies skin, promotes weight loss,
disinfects, reduces stress and arthritis, kills mold

Golden rod [**gohl**-duhn rod]

Treats kidney conditions and urinary issues,
antifungal, anti-inflammatory, relieves cold
symptoms

H

Hemp [hemp]

Antioxidant, improves cardiovascular condition, hydrates skin, lowers cholesterol, relieves diabetic symptoms

Hyssop [**his**-uhp]

Decongestant, astringent, antiseptic, increases circulation, relieves muscle spasms, aids in digestion

Honey [**huhn**-ee]

Antifungal, antioxidant, skin protectant, reduces allergy symptoms, increases energy, promotes weight loss, helps insomnia

Henna [**hen**-uh]

Used to treat ulcers, used for hair dying and other cosmetic purposes, anti-inflammatory, protects skin, relieves headaches and fevers

Helichrysum [hel-i-**krahy**-suhm]

> Treats skin disorders and conditions, antioxidant,
> anti-inflammatory, relieves digestive issues,
> helps insomnia

Horseradish [**hawrs**-rad-ish]

> Relieves cold and flu symptoms, helps digestive
> and urinary problems, antioxidant, pain reliever

J

Jojoba oil [hoh-**hoh**-buh oil]

> Moisturizes skin, promotes hair growth, anti-
> inflammatory, controls hair frizz

Jasmine [**jaz**-min]

> Soothing, builds confidence, increases your
> mood, aphrodisiac, antiseptic, fades scaring,
> curbs cravings and addictions

Juniper [**joo**-nuh-per]

Stimulating, relaxing, purifying, heals arthritis, astringent, helps with digestive issues

L

Lemongrass [**lem**-uhn-gras]

Toning, fortifying, insect repellent, relieves pain, astringent, detoxes body, treat insomnia, fights obesity

Lavender [**lav**-uhn-der]

Refreshing, soothing, promotes rest, heals skin conditions, toner, speeds up hair growth, relieves headaches

Lemon oil [**lem**-uhn oil]

Uplifting, antiseptic, repels insects, treats yeast infections, increases concentration, pain reliever

Lime oil [lahym oil]

Astringent, antiseptic, antiviral, treats

toothaches, relives diarrhea, increases appetite,

wrinkle reducer

M

Marjoram [**mahr**-jer-uhm]

Warming, sedative, improves digestion,

suppresses sexual desires, regulates menstrual

cycle, lowers blood pressure

Myrrh [mur]

Rejuvenating, fights mucus, relaxing, insect

repellent, prevents sunburn, antibacterial

Magnesium oil [mag-**nee**-zee-uhm oil]

> Relieves stress, reduces oil in skin, improves insomnia, aids in pain relief, relieves diabetes and high blood pressure symptoms

Mandarin [**man**-duh-rin]

> Improves skin, fights cancer causing cells, calms overactive children, helps with digestion, increases appetite

Melissa [muh-**lis**-uh]

> Treats insomnia, hypertension, diabetes, herpes, depression and dementia, antibacterial, relaxing, relieves menstrual problems

Mustard oil [**muhs**-terd oil]

> Regulates cholesterol levels, helps with digestion, combats cancer cells, relives numb muscles, controls cold symptoms

Myrtle [**mur**-tl]

Astringent, mild sedative, aphrodisiac, heals

hemorrhoid, relives allergy symptoms, treats

urinary infection

N

Neem [neem]

Cleanses and treats skin conditions, repels

parasites and insects, antifungal, skin toner,

promotes hair growth

Neroli [**neer**-uh-lee]

Relaxing, dispels fears, decreases swelling,

improves menopause symptoms, lowers blood

pressure

Nutmeg [**nuht**-meg]

Natural fragrance, helps with digestion, heightens concentration, used to treat bad breath, increases immunity

O

Olive oil [**ol**-iv oil]

Moisturizer, reduces wrinkles, treats high cholesterol, diabetes and dementia, promotes weight loss, relieves constipation

Orange oil [**or**-inj oil]

Refreshes, relaxing, repels insect, antiseptic, cleaning properties, relieves stress, increases circulation

Onion [**uhn**-yuhn]

Promotes hair growth, fights infections, pain

relief, increases cardiovascular health, treats

osteoporosis

Oregano [**uh**-reg-uh-noh]

Protect immune system, aids in digestion, boost

energy levels, treats osteoporosis, relives cold

symptoms

P

Peppermint [**pep**-er-mint]

Cooling, decongestant, treats digestive problems,

sharpens the mind, headache relief, increases

energy

Pine oil [pahyn oil]

Antiseptic, stimulating, increases immunity and

circulation in the body, relieve skin conditions

Patchouli oil [**pach**-oo-lee]

Helps fight depression and swelling, antiseptic,

treats dandruff and psoriasis, anti-inflammatory

Palo Santo [**pal**-oh **san**-toh]

Reduces swelling, increases immunity,

antibacterial, relives headaches, cold relief

Parsley [**pahr**-slee]

Regulates menstruation, reduces inflammation,

improves immunity, helps with digestion, fights

bad breath

Q

Quinoa [**keen**-wah]

High in protein and fiber, antioxidant, gluten

free, promotes weight loss, increase

cardiovascular health

R

Rose oil [rohz oil]

> Relaxing, enhances sexuality, astringent, treats anxiety, moisturizes dry skin, laxative

Rosemary [**rohz**-mair-ee]

> Invigorating, clarifying, improves memory, treats alopecia, relieves stress and pain

Roman chamomile [**roh**-muhn **kam**-uh-meel]

> Treats depression and PTSD, reduces stress, soothes irritated skin, relieves arthritis, lowers fevers

Rosewood [**rohz**-wood]

> Relieves headaches and tress, aphrodisiac, antiseptic, improves skin conditions, deodorizer, treats oral infections

Sesame oil [**ses**-uh-mee oil]

Improves dental and skin health, reduces

hypertension, high cholesterol and diabetes,

combats cancer cells, treats breathing issues

Sunflower oil [**suhn**-flou-er oil]

Combats cancer cells, high in protein, aids in

digestion, wrinkle reducer, light weight skin and

hair moisturizer, stops alopecia

Sage [seyj]

Slows down milk production, astringent,

wrinkle reducer, antidepressant, improves

memory, increases appetite

Shea butter [shey **buht**-er]

> Heavy skin and hair moisturizer, anti-inflammatory, wrinkle reducer, heals skin conditions

Sandalwood [**san**-dl-wood]

> Relaxing, warming, builds confidence, astringent, anti-inflammatory, heals wounds, increases memory

Sea salt [see sawlt]

> Relieves pain, detoxifies, exfoliates skin, relaxing, improves hair growth, reduces circles around the eyes

Spikenard [**spahyk**-nerd]

> Promotes hair growth, relaxing, repels fleas, increases immunity, treats insomnia, promotes fertility, helps with menstrual symptoms

Sea buckthorn oil [see **buhk**-thawrn oil]

Anti-inflammatory, relieves sunburns, prevents

infections, reduces diabetes symptoms

Savory [**sey**-vuh-ree]

Aphrodisiac, astringent, heals wounds and

intestinal problems, treats sore throat

Spearmint [**speer**-mint]

Clears congestion, aids with digestion,

antioxidant, treats insomnia, relieves pain

T

Turmeric [**tur**-mer-ik]

Anti-inflammatory, reduces tumors, fights

depression, relieves common cold symptoms,

treats wounds, gives skin a natural glow

Tea tree/Melaleuca [tee tree/mel-uh-**loo**-kuh]

> Antiseptic, strengthens immune system, kills
> mold, treats dandruff and respiratory issues

Thyme [tahym]

> Antiseptic, refreshes, strengthens immune
> system, aids in digestion, relieves respiratory
> issues

V

Vinegar [**vin**-i-ger]

> Great household cleaner, promotes weight loss,
> fights cancer cells, relieves pain, conditions hair

Vanilla [vuh-**nil**-uh]

> Natural fragrance, antioxidant, treats depression,
> anti-inflammatory, lowers fever and high
> cholesterol levels

Vitamin A [vahy-**tuh**-min ey]

Anti-inflammatory, increases eye sight, skin moisturizer, improves immunity, relieves measles symptoms

Vitamin E [vahy-**tuh**-min ee]

Antioxidant, promotes hair growth, hair and skin moisturizer, wrinkle reducer, cleanses skin

Vitamin D [vahy-**tuh**-min dee]

Improves bone health, increase muscle function, reduces diabetes issues, fights cancer cells

Vitamin K [vah-**tuh**-min key]

Can prevent cancer, diabetes and osteoporosis, increases blood clotting

Vetiver [**vet**-uh-ver]

Helps control ADHD and anxiety, treats heat exhaustion, boosts energy, increases circulation

Valerian [vuh-**leer**-ee-uhn]

Treats dementia, migraine pain and insomnia,

relives menstrual cramps, helps teeth grinding,

relaxing

W

Wintergreen [**win**-ter-green]

Relieves sore throats, helps with arthritis and

headaches, astringent, relaxing, eliminates odors

X

Xanthan gum [**zan**-thuhn guhm]

Sugar based natural thickener, fights cancer

cells

Xylitol [**zahy**-li-tawl]

Natural sweetener, improves oral health,

stabilizes pH in mouth, repair damaged tooth

enamel

Y

Ylang-ylang [**ee**-lahng-**ee**-lahng]

Relieves anxiety and depression, aphrodisiac, improves sleep, moisturizes dry skin, stimulates hair growth, increases circulation

Yarrow [**yar**-oh]

Lowers blood pressure levels, removes cold symptoms, treats insomnia and stress, relieves toothaches

Z

Zedoary [**zed**-oh-er-ee]

Helps wounds heal, purifies the blood, substitute for arrowroot, aphrodisiac

Write Your Own Recipes

Write Your Own Recipes

Write Your Own Recipes

Write Your Own Recipes

Write Your Own Recipes

Write Your Own Recipes

Supply List

Supply List

Notes

Notes

Conversion Chart

Measurement	Equivalent
1/16 teaspoon	dash
1/8 teaspoon	a pinch
3 teaspoons	1 tablespoon
1/8 cup	2 tablespoons
1/4 cup	4 tablespoons
1/3 cup	5 tablespoons plus 1 teaspoon
1/2 cup	8 tablespoons
3/4 cup	12 tablespoons
1 cup	16 tablespoons
1 Pound	16 ounces

US to Metric Conversions

Measurement	Equivalent
1/5 teaspoon	1 ml (ml stands for milliliter)
1 teaspoon	5 ml
1 tablespoon	15 ml
1 fluid oz.	30 ml
1/5 cup	50 ml
1 cup	240 ml
2 cups (1 pint)	470 ml
4 cups (1 quart)	.95 liter
4 quarts (1 gal.)	3.8 liters
1 oz.	28 grams
1 pound	454 grams

Raw Beauty Pledge

It's a pledge to remain physically active, consume healthier organic foods, use all-natural supplements, skin and hair care products, and seek spiritual and mental clarity!

There is no cost to join this movement! If you love it... We need you to help us spread this way of life! This movement can help us grow as individuals as well as strengthen broken communities! Together we can make phenomenal changes!!

To join the Raw Beauty Movement, you must make the conscious decision to use these 10 steps to improve your life daily!

1.	Participate in a physical activity for at least 30 minutes.

2.	Drive less miles and use fuel efficient transportation.

3.	Use more energy efficient appliances.

4.	Eat healthier Non-GMO organic foods.

5.	Use all-natural supplements, vitamins and enhancements.

6.	Use all-natural hair, skin and cleaning products.

7.	Wear less toxic organic clothing.

8.	Research everything!

9.	Seek spiritual wholeness.

10.	Sow a seed! (mentally, spiritually, or physically)